A
Cooperative
Method
of
NATURAL
BIRTH
CONTROL

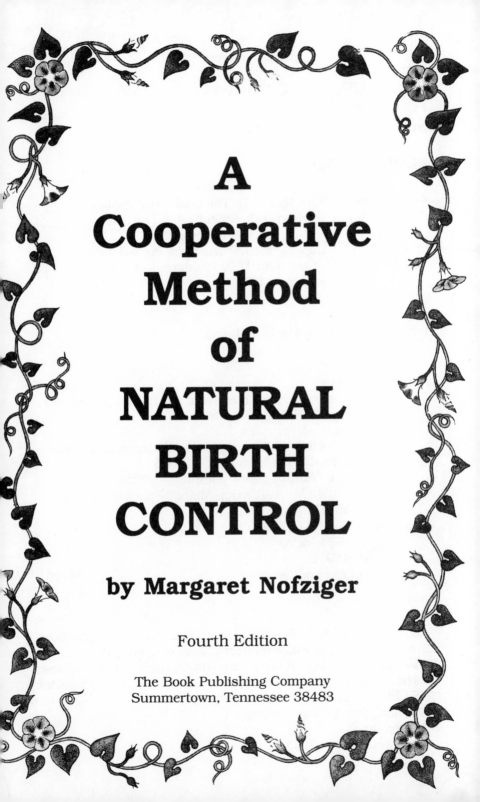

A Cooperative Method of NATURAL BIRTH CONTROL

by Margaret Nofziger

Fourth Edition

The Book Publishing Company
Summertown, Tennessee 38483

BOOK PUBLISHING COMPANY
PO Box 99
Summertown, TN 38483

ISBN 0-913990-84-1

First Edition -- Copyright 1976 The Book Publishing Co.
Second Edition, Revised -- Copyright 1978 The Book
                                    Publishing Co.
Third Edition -- Copyright 1979 The Book Publishing Co.
Fourth Edition -- Copyright 1992 Margaret Nofziger
                      First printing 1992
                      Second printing 1993

Front cover photo by David Frohman

Nofziger, Margaret.
            A cooperative method of natural birth control /
      by Margaret Nofziger. -- 4th ed.
                      p.   cm.
            Includes bibliographical references and index.
            ISBN 0-913990-84-1 : $6.95
            1. Natural family planning. I. Title.
            [DNLM: 1. Rhythm Method--popular works.
      WP 630 N773c]
      RG136.5.N64   1992
      613.9'434--dc20
      DNLM/DLC
      for Library of Congress   91-33429
                                                 CIP

Contents

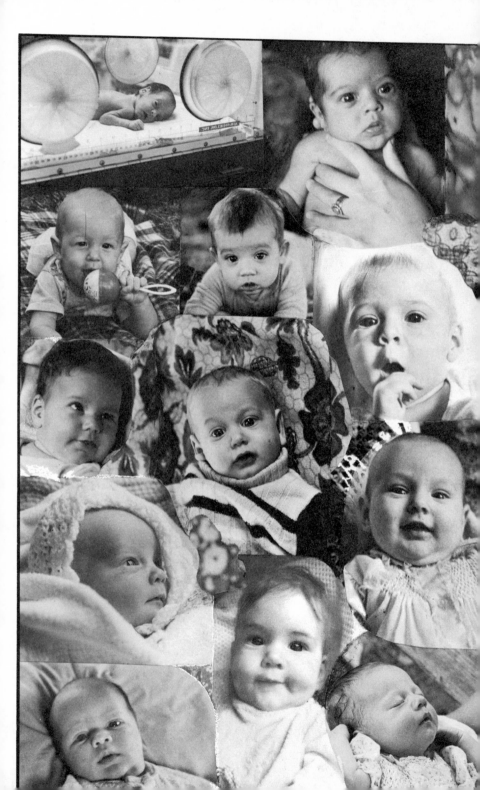

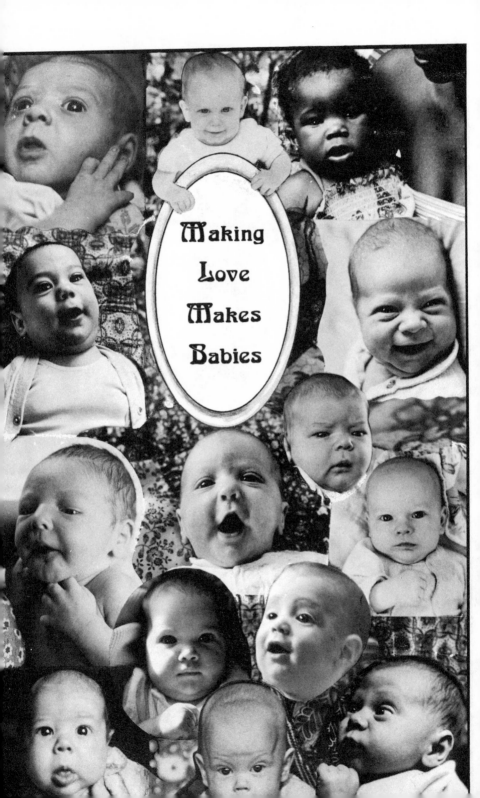

Making

Love

Makes

Babies

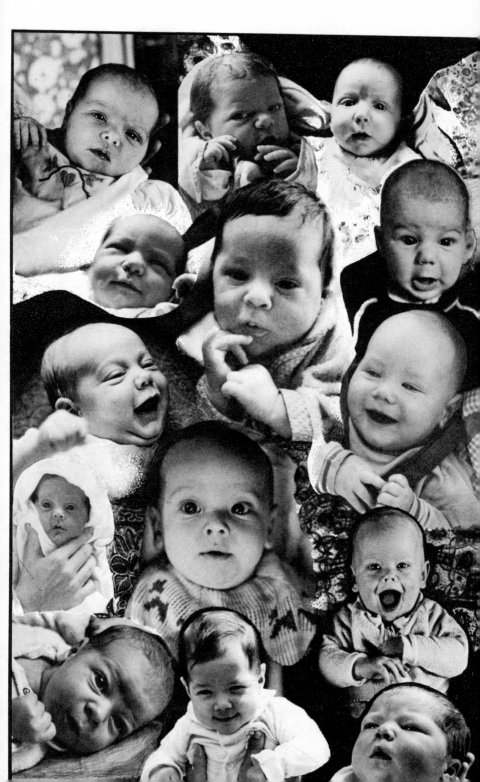

If you wish to avoid or postpone making babies, you could abstain from making love during those times when you might conceive. This book will help you find out when those fertile times occur.

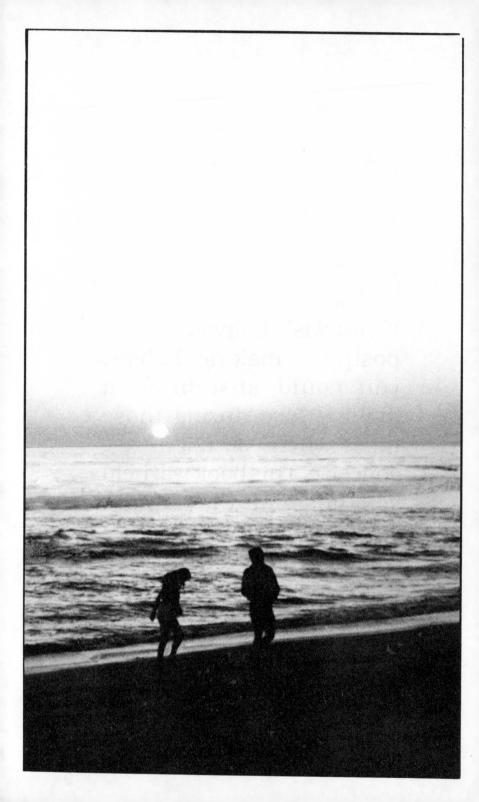

A Word For Love

I want to put in a word for love here, before we get into details of this method. This is the only form of birth control that is a *cooperative* venture. Neither husband nor wife has to bear a health burden or do it alone. It is the only non-sexist form of birth control, requiring the love and understanding of both.

The basis of this method is the *agreement* to pay close attention and lovingly abstain for a bit in order to not conceive at this time. This way, when you do make love, it is complete and open to all the life force energy there is. And when you are not prepared to conceive, you don't do what causes conception. Now, don't give up loving altogether. There are many ways to show your love besides the usual way. With love and imagination, those few days a month can be as fulfilling and repairing as the rest. Learning how to cooperate on this issue tends to draw a couple closer together.

Getting to Know Your Cycle

First let's take a close look at a time line of the fertility cycle of women and find out when ovulation is likely to occur. Most women ovulate about two weeks *before* their following period. (Not 14 days after the previous period.) It can happen anywhere from 12-16 days before, but mostly around 14 days before. A common mistake is the idea that ovulation takes place 14 days after your period, because people usually talk in terms of a 28 day cycle where it's 14 days either way. It makes quite a difference if your cycle is longer or shorter than 28 days.

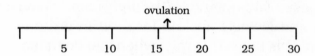

This is a 30 day cycle. Day 1 of the cycle is day 1 of the period. In this cycle, she would probably ovulate around the 16th day—14 days before her next period.

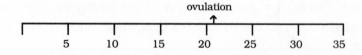

In this 35 day cycle, she ovulated around the 21st day.

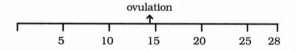

In this 28 day cycle, she ovulated around the 14th day.

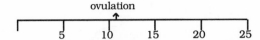

In this 25 day cycle, she ovulated around the 11th day.

As you can see from these different examples, the segment after ovulation is pretty constant—about 2 weeks. This is because when ovulation occurs and the egg bursts from the ovary, there is a hole or crater left where the egg was. This hole, the *corpus luteum*, becomes a hormone secreting gland and secretes *progesterone.* This gland has a *temporary lifespan* of approximately a fortnight, or 12-16 days. Then this gland heals over, the progesterone stops and the period commences. This limited, regular lifespan of the corpus luteum is the reason for the fairly constant length of the "after-ovulation" phase of the cycle. But the segment before ovulation will vary according to the length of the cycle.

The cycle goes through its changes because of hormones. Ordinarily, these hormones interact with each other to make the cycle change at an orderly pace each month. But some of these hormones are regulated by a part of the brain called the *hypothalamus*, and this part of the brain is influenced by outside factors such as health, travel, physical or mental stress, and upsetting emotions such as fear and anger or chronic anxiety.

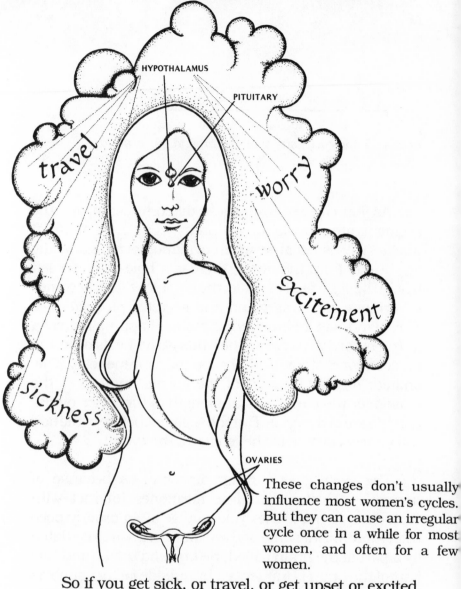

These changes don't usually influence most women's cycles. But they can cause an irregular cycle once in a while for most women, and often for a few women.

So if you get sick, or travel, or get upset or excited, this can make you have an unusually early or late ovulation, and then have an early or late period.

There are warning signs of early or late ovulation— the same cervical mucus changes that warn you of regular ovulation. But you must pay special attention when there is sickness or travel or stress in a cycle so that you don't miss the signals if they come before you expect them.

The Egg & The Sperm

In order for a pregnancy to occur, a fresh, live sperm from the man must meet and fertilize a live egg from the woman. This can only happen during a few days in a women's fertility cycle. Pregnancy can happen if you make love at the exact time of ovulation. You can also get pregnant by making loveup to 72 hours before or 24 hours after ovulation. This is because:

THE EGG ONLY LIVES FOR 12-24 HOURS
and
SPERM CAN FERTILIZE AN EGG FOR 2-3 DAYS [1]
(POSSIBLY UP TO 5)

So in order to avoid pregnancy, a couple needs to abstain from making love for 3 days preceding ovulation and 1 day after.

This would be very simple if we could pinpoint the exact time of ovulation. But at this stage of fertility research, we can only estimate the approximate time of ovulation and allow some extra leeway for error.

1. France JT. Biology of the fertile period.
   Int J Fertil 1981;26:143-152.

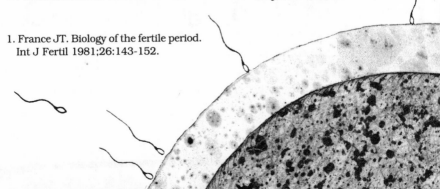

Female
Reproductive
Organs

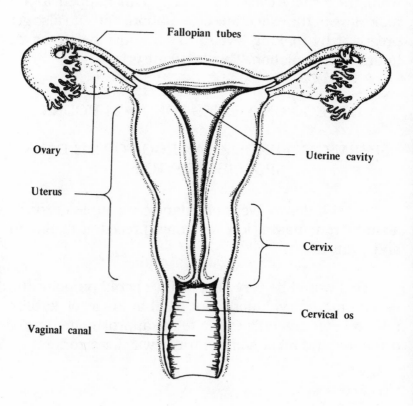

Fallopian tubes

Ovary

Uterus

Uterine cavity

Cervix

Cervical os

Vaginal canal

The Method
or
How to Do It

This method of natural birth control is actually three methods rolled into one. It is a combination of:

1. Charting your Basal Body Temperature (body-at-rest-temperature)

2. Calculating the early, pre-ovulatory infertile times with formulas from the rhythm system

and

3. Observing and charting the cervical mucus, which changes noticeably during the monthly cycle.

We will use the rhythm system for finding the infertile time before ovulation.

The Basal Body Temperature charting is for finding the safe, infertile time after ovulation. The mucus observation will anticipate an unexpected early ovulation, and will help confirm when ovulation has passed.

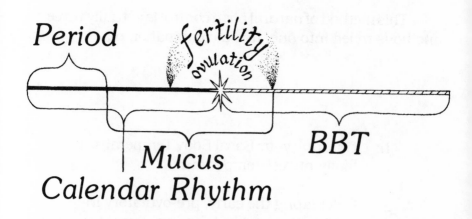

This method is called "natural" because it is based on recognizing the natural changes in a woman's fertility cycle, and avoiding intercourse on those days when she is fertile.

There are natural signs and symptoms that occur in a woman's body that can distinguish the different phases of her cycle, and especially the days surrounding ovulation.

Ovulation is when the egg bursts from its follicle in the ovary and travels toward the womb.

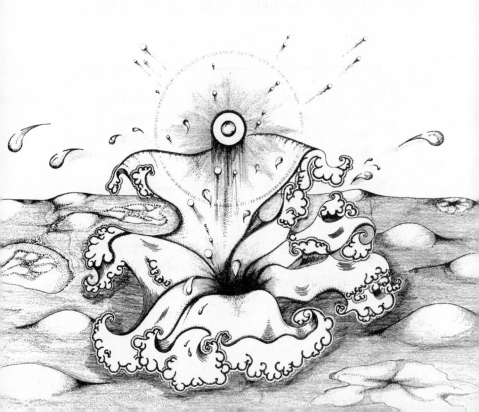

It is pretty easy to find out when you have already ovulated because your Basal Body Temperature—BBT—rises right after ovulation and stays up until a few days before your next period.

BUT IT IS TRICKIER TO FIND OUT WHEN OVULATION IS APPROACHING

You need to have 5 days warning so you won't have any sperm in the fallopian tube ready and waiting for the egg to burst from its follicle and come meet them.

> A calendar rhythm formula and careful mucus observation are the methods available for predicting the "safe," infertile days before ovulation.

We will talk about the early part of the cycle first to keep everything in order, but remember, the safest time of the cycle is after the BBT has shown that ovulation has already occurred.

> *To avoid pregnancy, the safest time to make love is after you are sure you have already ovulated.* It is easier to determine when ovulation *has already occurred* than it is to know when it *will happen.* The main way to know that ovulation has already happened is that *your basal temperature will rise noticeably after ovulation.*

If you want the absolutely surest, most infallible form of natural birth control, I would suggest what the French call "la methode dure," the strict method. This is where you only make love in the latter part of the cycle after the rise in temperature, and avoid intercourse during the time between the period and ovulation.

The strict temperature method is 98.6 - 99.2 % effective. [1] (Pearl index of .8 - 1.4 pregnancies per 100 woman years.) This statistic includes failures in application of the method.

1. World Health Organization, *Biology of Fertility Control by Periodic Abstinence.* Technical Report Series #360, Geneva, 1967.

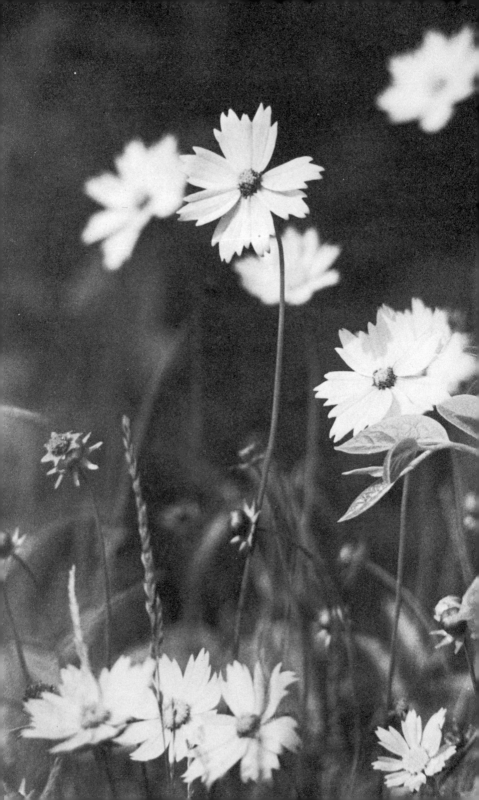

A Modified Rhythm

The first thing I want to say about calendar rhythm is:

CALENDAR RHYTHM ALONE IS NOT ENOUGH!!!

¡EL METODO DEL RITMO CALENDARIO SOLAMENTE NO ES BASTANTE!

KALENDAR RHYTHMUS ALLEIN GENÜGT NICHT!

LE RHYTHME D'APRÈS LE CALENDRIER TOUT SEUL NE SUFFIT PAS!

IL METODO DEL RITMO CALENDARIO SOLAMENTE NON BASTA!

DE KALENDER RHYTHME METHODE VOOR GEBOORTEBEPERKING IS NIET VOLDOENDE!

ATT FÖRLITA SIG PÅ "SÄKRA PERIODER" BESTÄMD MED ENBART ALMANACKAN RÄCKER INTE!

If you rely only on the rhythm method to avoid pregnancy, you may find yourself pregnant. Over the years, the rhythm method alone has proven to be only about 60 - 80 % effective.

Calendar Rhythm Method

The calendar rhythm method is one of the oldest means of determining times of fertility and infertility. It is a method based on the three physiological premises discussed in the previous chapter. These are:

> **(a)** Ovulation occurs approximately 2 weeks previous to the next period. Fourteen days is the average, but it can occur 12-16 days before the following period.
> **(b)** Sperm are usually viable (able to fertilize) for 3 days.
> **(c)** The lifespan of the egg (ovum) is 12-24 hours only.

So, if you had a list of your previous cycles for 12 months, or more (the more the better) you could subtract about 2 weeks from your very shortest cycles and find out approximately when you ovulated in these short cycles. This will tell you *the earliest you are likely to ovulate in future cycles.* Then you subtract about 2 weeks from the longest cycle you have experienced and this will tell you approximately when you ovulated on these long cycles; and therefore when it is *the latest you are likely to ovulate in future cycles.* To this estimated early observation day, you count back 2 more days in case you ovulate 16 days back from the next

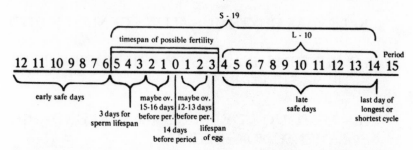

period instead of an even 2 weeks—14 days; and you count back 3 more days for the *lifespan of the sperm.* (Remember, sperm deposited 3 days previously can be ready and waiting at the time of ovulation.) This gives you your last safe infertile day *according to past history* of your cycles. To the cycle day of your latest past ovulation, you will add 2 days in case your ovulation precedes the next period by 12 days instead of an even 2 weeks, and then you add 1 more day to account for the 24-hour maximum lifespan of the egg. This gives you your first infertile day after the egg has come and gone, and establishes your late safe days. From this reasoning came the original calendar rhythm formulas, the most popular of which was Ogino's formula of:

Shortest minus 19 for early pre-ovulation safe days
and
Longest minus 10 for late, post-ovulation safe days.

Since we will use the temperature method to establish the late safe days after ovulation, we will not be concerned with the later half of the formula. There is no need to abstain allowing for one's longest possible cycle (therefore latest ovulation) in one's entire history when the temperature can establish the passing of fertility in each individual cycle. So, what we need from the calendar rhythm system is the concept of an "early safe days formula" based on the previous cycle patterns. The original Ogino formula of S - 19 has a very small, but nonetheless present, failure rate—in other words, a few pregnancies. So we will adopt a modified rhythm formula for early safe (infertile) days of:

S - 21 = last infertile day of the pre-ovulation phase.

This formula is intended to give you about 7 days leeway before your estimated time of ovulation (a fortnight before the coming period)—5 days for maximum sperm life and 2 more days in case you ovulate 16 rather than 14 days before your next period.

For Example:
If your shortest recorded cycle was 28 days, you would quit making love after day 7—fertility begins on day 8.

28-21 = 7, as the last safe day.

If your shortest recorded cycle was 32 days, you would quit making love after day 11—fertility begins on day 12.

32-21 = 11, as the last safe day.

Shortest Recorded Cycle	Last day Infertile	First day Fertile
25	4	5
26	5	6
27	6	7
28	7	8
29	8	9
30	9	10
31	10	11
32	11	12
33	12	13
34	13	14
35	14	15

This is more reliable the more past cycles you are considering. If you never had a cycle shorter than 28 days in the last several years, you could be pretty sure of infertility through day 7. But you still need to watch your mucus carefully in this early part of the cycle, or you could be in for a surprise.

When you begin using this method, you may not know the length of your shortest cycles. In this case, you can make love through day 5 of your cycles for the first six months, and then apply the formula.

*Remember: To find the number of days of your cycle, start with day 1 of your period, and go to the **number of the last day before your next period.***

IMPORTANT

Only use these days **if your mucus also says you're not fertile.** If any of these systems tell you that you are fertile, you'd better believe it!

REMEMBER: The calendar rhythm method alone is not really reliable enough for determining the early infertile days before ovulation because the day of ovulation can *occasionally be changed by illness, stress, travel, and drugs such as antibiotics and tranquilizers.* (These stresses can also affect the next cycle.) So you need to use your modified rhythm formula in conjunction with:

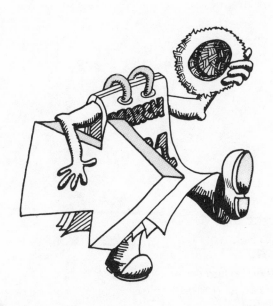

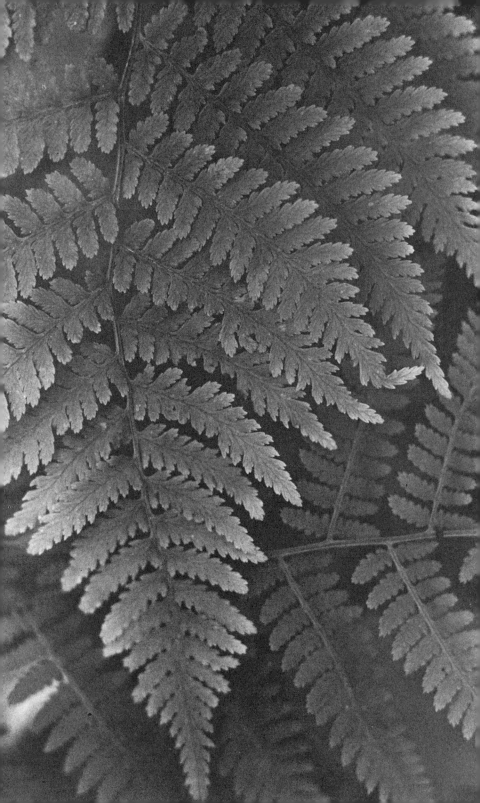

Cervical Mucus—
An Indicator of Fertility

In some cultures or situations, it is not practical to keep a BBT chart. In that case, the cervical mucus observation with an "early days" formula would be best if the temperature cannot be charted. It is far more accurate than calendar rhythm alone. But I strongly urge you to invest your time and energy in the COMBINATION METHOD, and use all the signs we have available to check.

If at all possible, you should use this mucus method of birth control along with a graph of your Basal Body Temperature, and a record of your past cycles.

You are creating cervical mucus all the time. It is produced by special cells up inside the cervix and changes character during the monthly cycle. You may have noticed this normal discharge and wondered why it was so profuse at times and absent at other times.

There are about 100 gland-like crypts producing cervical mucus.

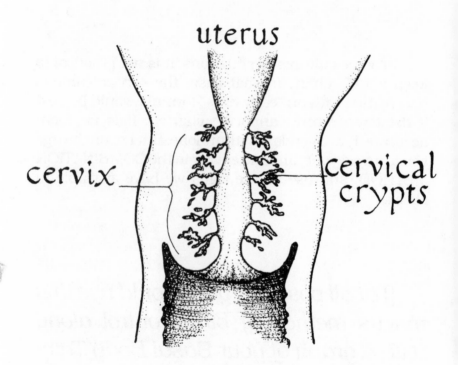

Many sperm find their way into the mucus-producing crypts, or caves, where they can be safely stored, fed, and gradually released upward over a period of hours or days.

The cyclic changes in your mucus discharge are controlled by the reproductive hormones.

In the beginning and end of the cycle, when the hormone **estrogen** is low, the mucus is scant, sticky and opaque with cellular matter. In the middle of the cycle, it changes to fertile type mucus. As the estrogen level increases, preparing for ovulation, the quantity of mucus *increases*. It becomes thinner and milkier. Then with more estrogen it gets clearer and more watery. At the estrogen peak, right before ovulation,it gets slick and glassy and you may be able to stretch an unbroken shimmering thread of it between your thumb and forefinger or between two slides.

At this fertile time, the mucus *has usually increased to ten times what it was earlier.* This abundant fertile mucus is helpful to sperm. It nourishes them, guides them upward through its fiber-like channels, protects them from the acid pH of your vagina (the mucus is alkaline), and keeps them from being swallowed up by phagocytes.*

After ovulation, the hormone **progesterone** causes the mucus to change to an infertile type within a day or two. Progesterone inhibits the mucus producing cells of the cervix and the mucus again becomes scant, thick, sticky, and opaque white or yellow from cellular matter and protein content. Infertile mucus, aside from indicating that you are not ovulating right now, also forms a thick criss-cross barrier across the cervix and keeps sperm and anything else from getting past the cervix into the womb for most of the cycle.

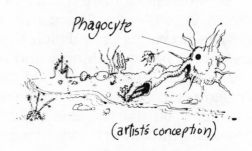

Phagocyte

(artist's conception)

*Phagocyte—a cell which has the ability to ingest and destroy substances such as bacteria, protozoa, cells, and cell debris.
—*Taber's Cyclopedic Medical Dictionary*

Macromolecules of Mucus— A Hydrogel

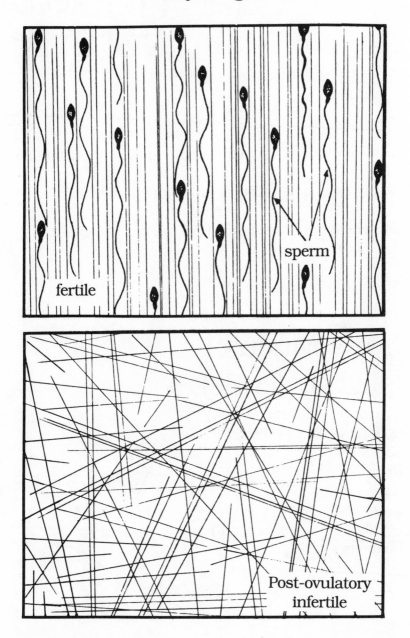

fertile

sperm

Post-ovulatory
infertile

Dry:

A little moist inside, but dry on the outside of your vagina.

No dripping or staining at all in your underwear.

No sensation of wetness, slipperiness, lubrication, discharge.

A sensation of dryness.

Early Mucus:
(slightly fertile)

opaque white or yellow
sticky
thick
pasty
tacky
cellular (dense matter in it)
holds its shape

Wet: Fertile

thin and watery
increasing amounts
translucent white or yellow
milky
cloudy
clear
acellular (no dense matter in it)
red, pink, or brown from blood (spotting)
liquid
flowing

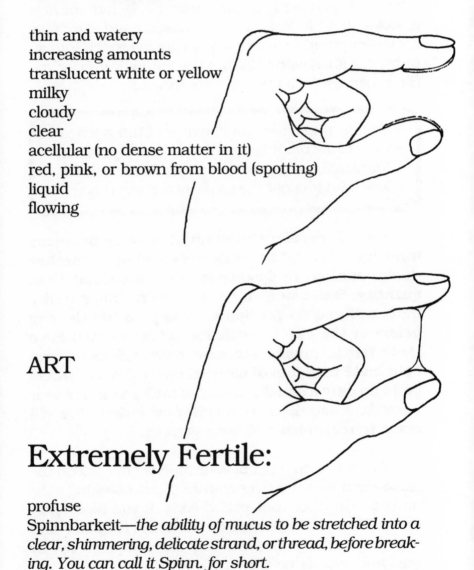

ART

Extremely Fertile:

profuse
Spinnbarkeit—*the ability of mucus to be stretched into a clear, shimmering, delicate strand, or thread, before breaking. You can call it Spinn. for short.*

35

To anticipate ovulation (and a few days before ovulation), **as an adjunct to your temperature graph and "early days" formula,** you will need to check your cervical mucus several times every day. You will find this mucus at your vaginal *opening*—you do not need to check inside. Check it after you have been up out of bed for a bit, but before you bathe or shower. Before you use the toilet is another good time to check. Determine how it looks, how it feels in your vagina, and check its consistency and *Spinnbarkeit* (ability to stretch into an unbroken fiber) with your first finger and thumb (or you can observe it on a piece of toilet tissue.)

> You need to check your mucus at times when you are not ready to make love. You will produce lubricating mucus when you are about to make love, and it is not the same as cervical mucus.

There is usually a substantial increase in mucus from dry to "early" to fertile to extremely fertile; but *don't count on it.* Quality is more important than quantity. Some women never see extremely fertile mucus. If you do get Spinn., it is probably the day before or the day of ovulation. Some women have their fertile mucus increase over 4-5 days, and culminate with lots of clear, slippery Spinn. Others build up only a small amount of milky wetness over a few days and then dry up after ovulation. You will come to recognize your own pattern.

You can keep track of your mucus changes on the same chart as your temperature. Start checking your mucus right after your period ends. If you have short cycles, 25 days or less, check it on the last couple of days of your period. The flow will be scant and pretty dry by then and will not be slippery unless there is *also some fertile mucus.*

So, first you establish your "early safe days" with S-21,

then you check this supposed safe time against your mucus observation. If you are anything but dry during the "safe time", your mucus may be warning you of an **unexpected early ovulation,** so you must consider that the fertile phase has begun and abstinence becomes necessary.

Usually the first few days after your period are

-- Noticeably Dry --

1	2	3	4	5	6	7	8	9	10	11	12	13
period	period	period	period	period	dry	dry	dry					

This dry time is not fertile unless it is considered fertile according to S-21.

During the dry days, it is a good idea to make love only at night after a full day's observations and also only *every other dry night* because you will probably be wet on the day following making love and unable to determine the condition of your mucus. Later on when you are experienced, you could stop skipping a day *only if you always lose* **all** *seminal fluid before noon and the remainder of the day is dry.*

Once the mucus has begun, it will probably be of the thick, sticky, "early" type. This mucus is not nearly as fertile as the wet mucus or Spinn. but it may have a few open channels to the cervix (where the sperm can be nourished and protected) so it too must be considered potentially fertile.

Next you will observe the

-- Wet, Fertile Mucus --

1	2	3	4	5	6	7	8	9	10	11	12	13	14	15	16	17	18
period	period	period	period	period	dry	dry	dry	sticky	sticky	creamy	milky	milky	clear wet	spinn			

usually culminating with the extremely fertile, stretchy Spinn. (Sometimes this is merely a *slick sensation* at your vaginal opening.)

Fertile mucus leads up to ovulation and will be primarily wet. It can be milky white, translucent yellow or clear. It can also be tinged pink or brown as there is sometimes a little breakthrough bleeding at the time of ovulation. *The consistency and color will go through changes as the fertile mucus builds up toward ovulation, which takes anywhere from 1-6 days or more.*

Do not make love after the appearance of any type of mucus because the smooth creamy kind can change to the wet kind very quickly.

Don't wait to see the mucus. If you *feel* a slippery or dripping sensation, it doesn't matter if you can see or collect any or not. Quality is more important than quantity.

The last day of this fertile (sometimes extremely fertile) mucus is the most fertile day of the cycle and is usually either the day of or the day before ovulation. The day before ovulation is very fertile because you can make love on this day and have the sperm ready and waiting for the egg to emerge.

Any mucus means ovulation may be approaching.

38

Fertile type mucus is also noted by its ability to "fern", that is to form fern-like patterns when it is dried on a slide. If you have a microscope, you can look at it. This ferning is caused by a higher salt content during the height of mucus production.

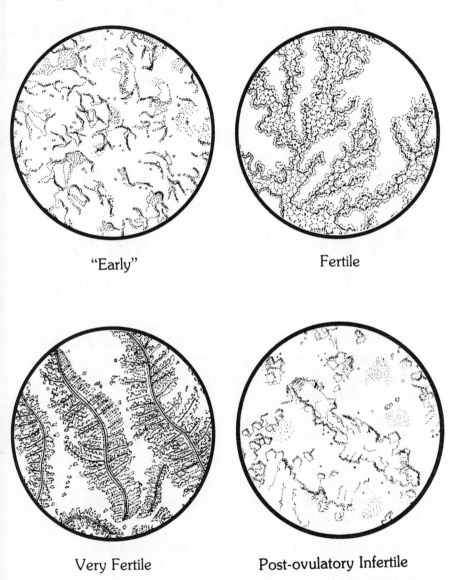

"Early"

Fertile

Very Fertile

Post-ovulatory Infertile

After the fertile phase, the mucus will return to the dry or sticky type.

1	2	3	4	5	6	7	8	9	10	11	12	13	14	15	16	17	18	19	20
period	period	period	period	period	dry	dry	dry	sticky	sticky	creamy	milky	milky	clear wet	spinn	sticky	tacky	dry	dry	dry

The 4th day* after it dries up, you are no longer fertile.

[This should correspond to the 3rd day of higher temps.]

Remember, if your mucus says you are infertile, and your temperature says you are fertile, wait. If your temperature says you are infertile and your mucus says you are still fertile, wait.

Don't ever play one system against the other. Use the most conservative data from each system.

(One exception: If your mucus gets a little milky later in the month, after it has demonstrated ovulation, *and your temperature is still up*, it's OK—not fertile.)

*For the vast majority of women, any time during the 4th day is safe. But if you want the utmost in surety, you can add the extra 12 hours and wait until evening.

If you have long cycles, and therefore a long pre-ovulatory phase, you may show some mucus before the true pre-ovulatory mucus build-up. If you have some mucus earlier than you expect it for ovulation, abstain for its duration and for 3 days after it. Then you can go back to making love every other dry night until your rhythm S-21 tells you to stop.

After your temperature and mucus have both demonstrated that ovulation has passed by two days, you can resume making love, every day if you wish, until the end of the cycle.

Any mucus you have from now on is not fertile. **Once ovulation has been established by both your temperature and your fertile mucus, and your temperature *remains high,*** you are infertile, even if you have some sticky or cloudy mucus later in the cycle. Also, it is very common to have a temperature drop and some wet mucus for a few days before your next period. This does not mean you are fertile, just that your period is coming. It is caused by hormone changes.

Special reminder: On the days when you're supposed to abstain, don't make love using withdrawl. One drop on the outside of your vagina can get you pregnant, and your man could lose a drop before he knows it.

Special reminder #2: If you have a yeast infection— itching and burning, or any other vaginal infection, don't make love until it is cleared up. Making love will make it worse, and most important, you will not get an accurate mucus reading.

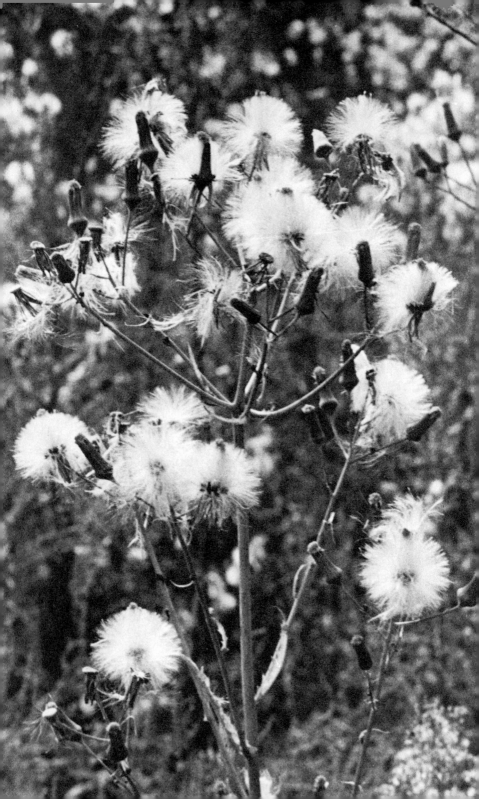

Basal Body Temperature

The cyclic changes in a woman's Basal Body Temperature form the mainstay of this combination method of natural birth control. A reproductive hormone that is released after ovulation causes the Basal Body Temperature to rise several tenths of one degree over what it was before ovulation.

TO AVOID PREGNANCY, THE SAFEST TIME TO MAKE LOVE IS AFTER YOU ARE SURE YOU HAVE ALREADY OVULATED.

It is easier to determine when ovulation *has already occurred* that it is to know when it *will happen.* The main way you know that ovulation has already happened is that:

YOUR BASAL TEMPERATURE WILL
RISE NOTICEABLY AFTER OVULATION

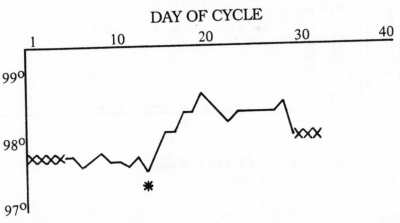

YOUR BASAL BODY TEMPERATURE IS THE TEMPERATURE OF YOUR BODY AT COMPLETE REST.

You take your temperature each morning and record it on a graph and connect each dot with a line. You will get a curve that begins low in the early part of the cycle and rises at, or right after, ovulation.

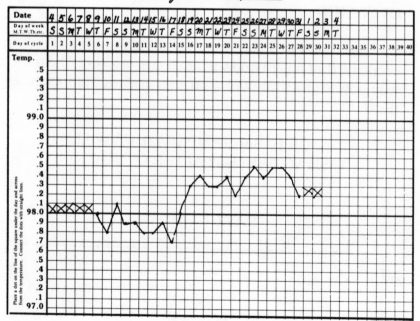

BASAL TEMPERATURE AND MUCUS CHART

MONTH *August* thru *September*

Put the dot on the line of the square that is below the day, and to the right of the correct temperature.

You can find your BBT with a special kind of thermometer called a Basal Thermometer. A Basal Thermometer is different from a regular fever thermometer because it records just the degrees of 95 to 100 and has a mark for each 1/10th of a degree.

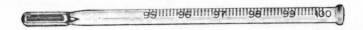

Basal thermometer

A regular fever thermometer records from 94 to 108 and has a mark for every 2/10 of a degree.

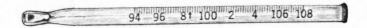

Regular thermometer

I suggest you invest in a Basal Thermometer (ask your druggist) because it is easier to read in the wee morning hours and is accurate to 1/10 of a degree. You can also use a digital electronic thermometer, which measures single tenths of a degree.

HOW TO READ YOUR MERCURY THERMOMETER

To read your temperature on your thermometer, hold it near a good light, and turn it slowly until you can see a shiny silver line (mercury) that goes from the silver bulb to part way out the numbers and lines.

The numbers represent whole degrees and the lines between the numbers represent parts of that whole degree.

Basal Thermometer

With a basal thermometer, look at the number which the mercury (silver line) has already passed. That is the number of whole degrees. Next, count each small line which the mercury has passed. This number of small lines is the number of 1/10 degrees. You express the 1/10 degrees by saying "point six" for six-tenths (6/10). You say "point two" for two-tenths (2/10) of a degree. Here are some examples:

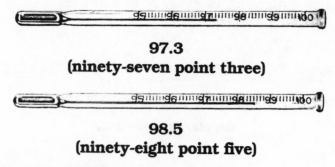

97.3
(ninety-seven point three)

98.5
(ninety-eight point five)

Regular Thermometer

If you are using a regular fever thermometer, count each small line that the mercury has passed as 2/10 of a degree instead of 1/10 of a degree. Count by "twos" for each small line: two-tenths, four-tenths, six-tenths, etc. Another difference is that the fever thermometer only has numbers for every other number—the even numbers. It has a lot more degrees on the glass tube than a basal thermometer, and doesn't have room for each whole number. The odd numbers are shown by a tall line.

The tall line between 94 and 96 is for 95. The tall line between 96 and 98 is for 97. The shorter lines represent two-tenths (2/10) of a degree each.

95.4 96.6 99.8

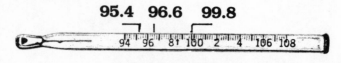

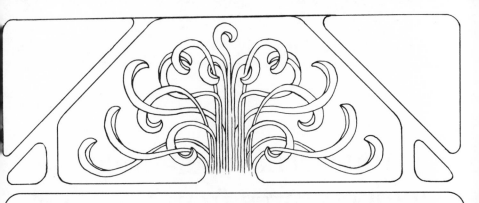

BBT INSTRUCTIONS

Take your temperature every morning after at least four hours of sleep and before getting out of bed, eating, or drinking. (Shake your thermometer down the night before.) You should take your temperature rectally or vaginally rather than in your mouth because it is more accurate, and accuracy is certainly what we need. Don't ever take it orally one half of the month and rectally or vaginally the other half because there is about a degree difference between the two. Don't wash the thermometer in hot water. Just wipe it with alcohol or use probe covers.

A very important aspect of this method is keeping good charts and records. Write your temperature on a graph to make a curve you can look at. It won't do to just write some numbers on your calendar. You won't be able to see what's happening. Write your mucus changes down on the same chart. You will be glad you did when you can compare several months of charts and see exactly how your mucus lined up with your temperature. Put a lot of value in your charts. Keep them neat and clear to read. This is like taking a course in YOU. You are studying your body at a very detailed level, and should study it as carefully as you would a scientific course.

WARNING: When taking your temperature with a glass mercury thermometer, hold it securely so that it does not travel into the rectum, vagina or urethra.

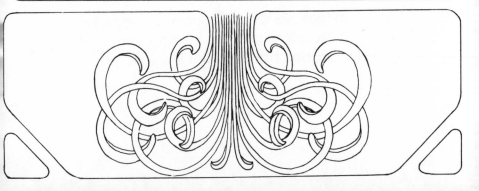

You will have relatively low temperatures from the time of your period until you ovulate. Ovulation will cause a rise of about 6/10th of one degree: .6° F.*, or six lines on your graph. This rise can happen in a day or it can stair-step up over a period of several days.

Ovulation took place right before the rise (sometimes characterized by a dip in temperature) or anywhere during the rise from low to high.

*.3°C.

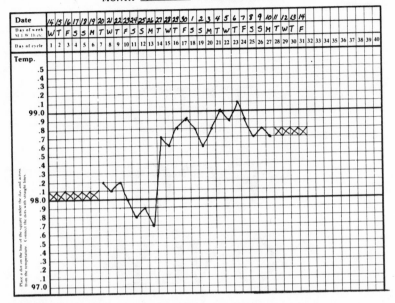

Sharp Rise

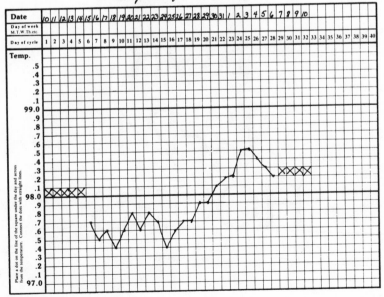

Stair-step Rise

THE EGG ONLY LIVES FOR 12-24 HOURS.

So, to avoid pregnancy, you want to avoid making love until the temperature has been in the high range for:

3 FULL DAYS

But sometimes it is difficult to tell what constitutes a rise, since it can happen abruptly or take several days to get to the high range.

So turn the page for an important rule to establish when the shift from low to high takes place.

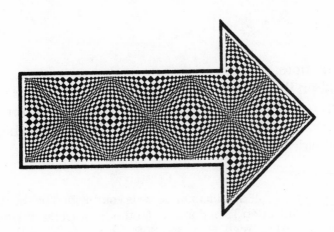

Don't make love until you have re-corded three consecutive temperatures that are .4°F (.2°C) higher than your temperatures for the six days previous to the rise. [1]

This means that when you start counting 1,2,3 - the day you call 1 must be .4° higher than the 6 days before the rise began, and it must stay .4 higher for days you call 2 and 3.

You can start making love again on the evening of day 3.

If this rule is difficult for you to use because your BBT does not make a clear and abrupt rise, use "Dr. Vollman's Rule" on p.55.

Mucus note:
If, on the day you would call "1", you still have some Spinn. type mucus, or if you still have maximum wet-ness, wait until the Spinn. is gone or the wetness begins to subside before counting "1".

1.The criteria for a "significant rise" was established by the World Health Organization Task Force on Methods for Determination of the Fertile Period (Tech. Rep. Ser. 360, 1968).

BASAL TEMPERATURE AND MUCUS CHART

MONTH _March_ thru _April_

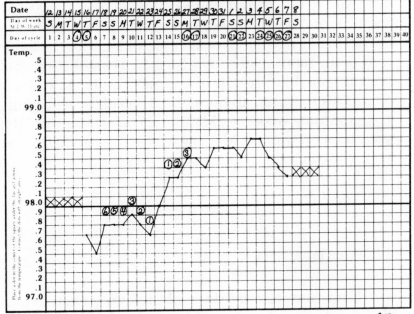

Number of days in this cycle: _27_
Shortest previous cycle: _27_

You can start taking your temperature each month on the 6th day unless you have short cycles under 25 days. In that case, take it from the first day of your period. After you've taken your temperature all month for a few months, and if your cycles are regular (less than 3 days variation in length,) you could quit taking it for the latter part of the month, after the rise is well established, and resume on the 6th day of the next cycle. Take your temperature within an hour and a half of the same time each morning upon awakening. If you sleep extra late, your temperature could show a false rise, so mark it on your chart.

Remember:

Your temperature does not tell you when ovulation is coming. It only tells you when it is done. *The safe times to make love before ovulation are a little more complicated to determine. To find out which early days are infertile before ovulation, if any, you use a rhythm formula of S-21 and observe your mucus for an early appearance which would indicate early fertility.*

If you have long cycles, and therefore a long pre-ovulatory phase, you may show some mucus before the true pre-ovulatory build-up. If you have some mucus earlier than you expect it for ovulation, abstain for its duration and until the night of the 4th dry day after it. Then you can go back to making love every other dry night until your rhythm S-21 tells you to stop.

Dr. Vollman's Rule

"I have used this rule now for 42 years, 656 couples with more than 32,000 menstrual cycles, 7 unplanned pregnancies, all from coitus in the postmenstrual phase."

-Rudolph Vollman, M.D.
Switzerland, April 1979

Dr. Vollman's temperature rule is a good one for women who have a slow rise or stairstep rise of their temperature. There have been no pregnancies due to the application of this rule. The 7 unplanned pregnancies he reports resulted from making love in the first part of the cycle, before ovulation, and before the temperature rise. (Dr. Vollman used an early days formula of *Shortest minus 20* for the last infertile day before ovulation.)

1. Add up all temperatures from the previous month (day 6 through the end). Calculate an *average* of these temperatures (to the 100th of a degree: 98.46).
2. Draw a line across the new chart at that average temp from the previous chart. If the average is 98.46, draw your line between 98.4 and 98.5.
3. Wait to make love until after you have recorded 4 temps *above that line*. If your average line is between, for instance, 98.4 and 98.5, you must reach 98.5 to be above the line. *The 4th morning is safe.*

See p. 70-72 for an example of "Dr. Vollman's rule".
(don't try to use this rule without studying the example.)

- If the temp drops .1°F below the line, skip that day in the count, but continue the count the next day.

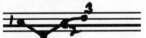

- If the temp drops more than .1°F below the line, start your count over.

- When calculating the average, do not add in and average any temp that is an obvious fever, or one that varies .8° - .9°F above or below the usual average.

About Fevers

Very, Very Important

If you get a fever, this will give you a *false high temperature reading.* Do not use this false high reading as proof that ovulation has passed. This could get you pregnant. A fever does not have to be 101.3 or 102 degrees to be a fever. A cold or flu virus would have no trouble raising your temperature two or three tenths of a degree. This may not be noticeable to you as a fever, but it would be enough to indicate a *false* high temperature on your chart. If you are sick, note it on your chart and don't trust any high temperatures. Abstain from making love until you are sure your fever has been gone for three days. Then evaluate your chart carefully. If you have any doubt at all, wait a little longer.

Remember also that any sickness can cause an early or late ovulation in this cycle and the next one, so be very careful.

Special reminder: On days when you're supposed to abstain, don't make love using withdrawal. One drop of semen on the outside of your vagina can get you pregnant, and your man could lose a drop even before he knows it.

MISSED PERIOD—If your period is late, don't assume that you are pregnant and quit practicing your birth control. You may have had a late ovulation which would result in a late period. Look at your temperature chart to see if your temperature rise took place later than usual. If it did, you could look for your period about two weeks after the rise. If the temperature remains high for over three weeks, you are probably pregnant.

A NOTE TO MEN

This method of natural birth control is called "cooperative" because it requires love and cooperation to work. You and your partner are assuming responsibility for your combined fertility. During some of her monthly cycle, you will need to abstain from intercourse. This is your chance to demonstrate, beyond words, your total love for your mate. Let her know that you love her through and through regardless of whether or not you can physically make love. You can help her keep track and chart, or you can leave it up to her and just trust her to tell you what's happening. Don't pressure her at all. Assure her it's OK with you if it's not a safe time. Remember, this is the safest way you can regulate your combined fertility. Following this method gracefully is an expression of love and will mature your relationship.

EXAMPLE CHARTS

This woman probably ovulated around day 14. Her first higher temperature wasn't high enough to call "number 1". The next day it rose more and this temperature was high enough to be called "1" (at least .4 ° higher than 6 temperatures before the rise.) On the 3rd day of higher temperatures, she was infertile for the remainder of the cycle.

BASAL TEMPERATURE AND MUCUS CHART

MONTH *April* thru *May*

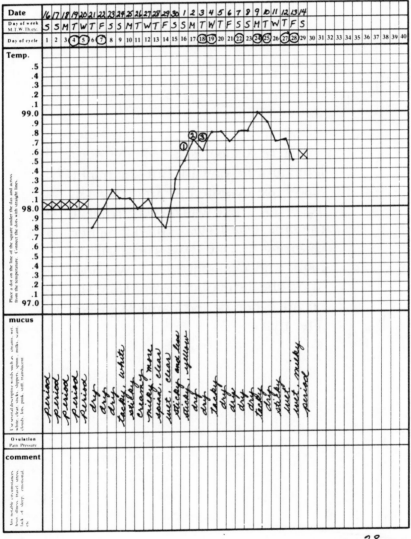

Number of days in this cycle: _28_

Shortest previous cycle: _28_

In retrospect, she probably ovulated around day 14, but she might also have ovulated around day 15, 16, or 17. There was no way to tell at the time. Day 18 was still not higher than day 13. Day 19 was finally truly high, and designated "1". We now know she did ovulate around day 14, because her period came 2 weeks after that.

BASAL TEMPERATURE AND MUCUS CHART

MONTH *June* thru *July*

Date	18	19	20	21	22	23	24	25	26	27	28	29	30	1	2	3	4	5	6	7	8	9	10	11	12	13	14	15	16											
Day of week M.T.W.Th.etc	S	S	M	T	W	T	F	S	S	M	T	W	T	F	S	S	M	T	W	T	F	S	S	M	T	W	T	F	S											
Day of cycle	1	2	③	④	⑤	6	7	8	9	10	11	12	13	14	15	16	17	18	19	20	21	㉒	23	㉔	㉕	㉖	27	㉘	29	30	31	32	33	34	35	36	37	38	39	40

Temp.

Place a dot on the line of the square under the day and across from the temperature. Connect the dots with straight lines.

.5
.4
.3
.2
.1
99.0
.9
.8
.7
.6
.5
.4
.3
.2
.1
98.0
.9
.8
.7
.6
.5
.4
.3
.2
.1
97.0

mucus

Use several descriptive words such as: creamy, wet, white, clear, sticky, slippery, sperm, milky, scant, cloudy, lots, pink, stiff, translucent.

period, period, period, period, dry, dry, dry, tacky – yellow, tacky – white, creamy – white, moist slippery, wet slippery, very wet, wet, scant sticky, very little, oily, milky, dry, dry, tacky, dry, tacky, dry, wet, wet, wet slippery, period

Ovulation Pain/Pressure

comment

Any notable circumstances: fever, illness, travel, stress, lack of sleep, emotional, etc.

travel, travel, travel, backache – AM.

Number of days in this cycle: __27__
Shortest previous cycle: __26__

61

This woman has very long cycles.* This one was 42 days long with ovulation around day 29. A lot of women would be having their period by day 29. She has to go by mucus and calendar rhythm for most of her cycle because ovulation and the temperature rise come so late in her cycle. Notice she didn't make love from day 13 through 16 because she had some early fertile looking mucus on day

13. After three dry days she resumed. She always stops making love by day 19 because her shortest recorded cycle was 40 days.

*As she gets older, her cycles will probably shorten, so she can't assume they will always be long.

BASAL TEMPERATURE AND MUCUS CHART

MONTH *January* thru *March*

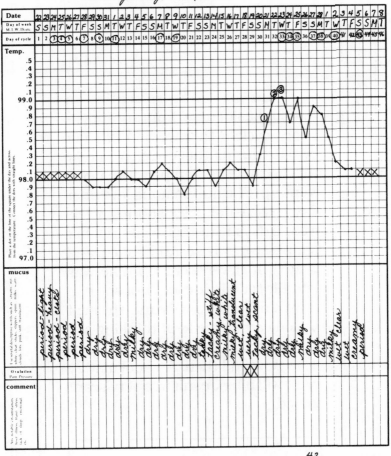

Number of days in this cycle: 42

Shortest previous cycle: 40

This is what is called a "monophasic curve" from an "anovulatory cycle". This woman did not ovulate during this cycle. We know this because her temperature never went up. She quit making love after day 8 as usual. (Her shortest cycle was 29 days.) She then waited for her temperature to rise. And waited, and waited. It never went up. She was infertile the whole cycle, but she had no way of knowing this until the next period came. She kept thinking she was just late ovulating. This happens now and then. An anovulatory cycle will often result in a very scant period.

Do not make love during or after the bleeding following a "monophasic curve" because it could be "breakthrough bleeding" of a late ovulation. It is safest to wait until after the temperature rise, whenever it comes.

BASAL TEMPERATURE AND MUCUS CHART

MONTH *April* thru *May*

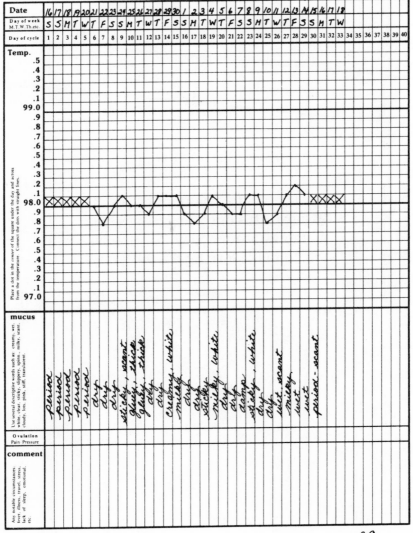

Number of days in this cycle: 29

Shortest previous cycle: 29

This woman has long cycles: 33-36 days. This one was 35 days, with ovulation around day 20. She was able to make love by the 24th day.

BASAL TEMPERATURE AND MUCUS CHART

MONTH *August* thru *September*

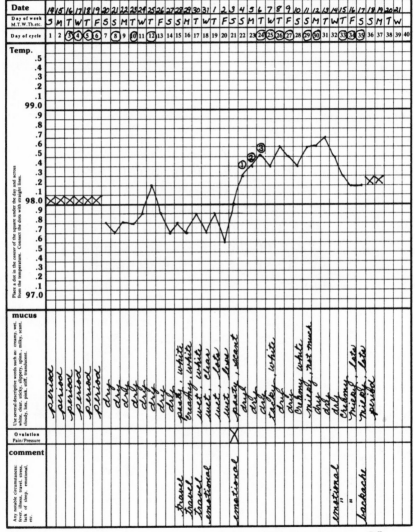

Number of days in this cycle: **35**

Shortest previous cycle: **33**

This woman has very long cycles of 39-45 days. Often she can make love through day 18 (39 - 21 = 18) because she is usually quite dry until then. This month she had some wet mucus on day 11, so she abstained for three days and then resumed on day 15.

BASAL TEMPERATURE AND MUCUS CHART

MONTH *September* thru *October*

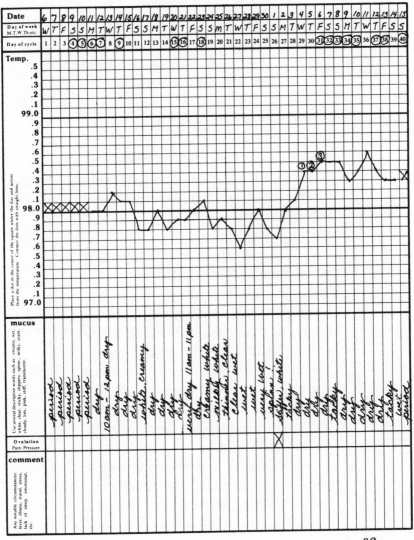

Number of days in this cycle: _39_
Shortest previous cycle: _39_

Dr. Vollman's Rule

This woman uses Dr. Vollman's rule. She has a gradual rise, and it doesn't usually have a .4° difference between the early lows and the highs after ovulation. She averaged her temperatures from the 5th day through the 27th day:

Last month, her average temperature was 98.29. She drew a line between 98.2 and 98.3 on this month's chart. Her temperature will need to reach at least 98.3 to be above the line. By the 19th day, she had recorded 4 temperatures above the line. (Remember, with Dr. Vollman's rule you are infertile on the 4th day of high temperature, not on the 3rd night.)

This month, her average temperature was 98.28, so herline remains about the same for the next month.

BASAL TEMPERATURE AND MUCUS CHART

MONTH *July* ___ thru *August*

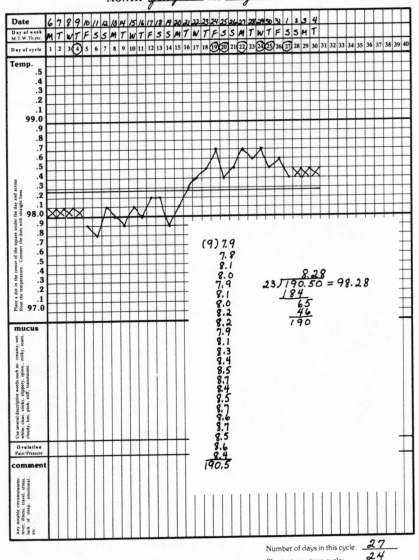

Number of days in this cycle: **27**

Shortest previous cycle: **24**

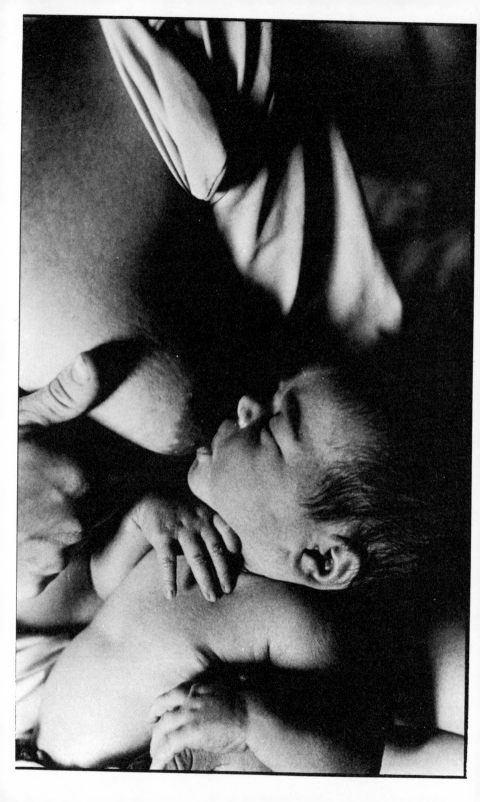

Mucus Method
For Nursing Mothers
With No Periods

Your periods can resume, and fertility with them, any time after the birth of your child. A lot of women don't get that first period until a month or two after weaning, but a substantial number get their period within a couple of months after delivery.

It is true that you are not fertile for most of the time that you are not having periods. But you cannot tell when your first period will come, and

OVULATION CAN TAKE PLACE BEFORE YOUR FIRST PERIOD.

So, since fertility can return shortly before the first period, you need to watch carefully for the fertile mucus that will come before your first ovulation.

To BBT or Not To BBT

It is up to you whether to chart your BBT while nursing or wait until you resume your cycles. There are advantages and disadvantages to charting your temperature before your periods return.

If you are breastfeeding, you could easily chart your temperature for nine months or a year before seeing a rise indicating the passing of ovulation. Breastfeeding makes you less likely to ovulate, especially if the baby nurses often, day and night, and receives no supplementary food. While you are not ovulating, your temp will be low, but may jump around. This kind of record could be discouraging and confusing for some women. On the other hand, it could be reassuring to see if the temperature went up after some fertile looking mucus or spotting, or stayed low. You could take your temperature every day or every few days, to see if it is staying low. And you could especially take it during times of mucus or spotting. Other than that, you could just chart your mucus.

A lot of nursing mothers resume their periods before total weaning, but some don't get their periods until a month or two after weaning. If you are only charting your mucus for the nursing time and still don't have periods at the time of weaning, you should start charting your temperature at this time.

If you wait until the first period to begin temperature

charting, you will not be able to make love during that first period. Without a temperature record showing some high temps before the bleeding, you can't know if it's a real period or "breakthough bleeding" of ovulation. If it were the latter, you would have no record of high temps before the first so-called period. You would then need to begin recording the temp and wait for a rise before making love.

If you had been taking your temp before the first bleeding, and the temps were high before it, you would know it was a period, and you could make love for the first four days of it. Then you should wait for a rise indicating the next ovulation has passed, before making love again.

A good "middle time" to begin taking your temperature is when you start adding solids to baby's diet, or when baby begins sleeping most or all of the night. When you start feeding baby any food besides breastmilk, or when baby sleeps many hours at a time, your breasts may not get enough stimulation to keep the hormones high which delay ovulation, and ovulation is more likely to happen. (Nursing delays ovulation for most women, but some women resume ovulation and periods early, even when breastfeeding often.)

If you are already taking your temp at the time of your first ovulation, you can confirm your mucus findings with the high temps which follow ovulation. Then, when you get your period, you will know it is really a period.

MUCUS METHOD—

Read the chapter on "Cervical Mucus—An Indicator of Fertility."

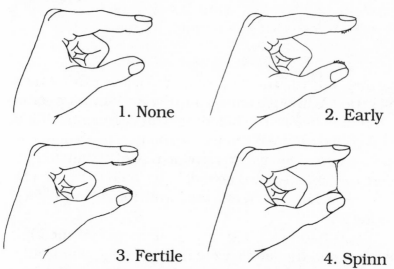

1. None
2. Early
3. Fertile
4. Spinn

Make love only on days when there is a definite *sensation of dryness* around the opening of your vagina.

During the dry days it is a good idea to make love only at night after a full day's observations and also only *every other dry night* because you will probably be a little wet on the following day, and unable to check the condition of your mucus.

If you show *one* day of mucus, abstain for that day and the following three dry days. The 4th dry day is infertile.

①	2	③	4	⑤	6	⑦	8	⑨	10	11	12	13	14	⑮	16
dry	–	*dry*	–	*dry*	–	*dry*	–	*dry*	–	*＊ wet ＊*	*dry*	*dry*	*dry*	*dry*	

Most women are quite dry for at least the first couple of months after childbirth (after cessation of the lochia). If there is any mucus at all, it is quite stiff and dry itself, not at all creamy or wet. This stiff, scant discharge can be considered "dry" if it is constant and unchanging in its character. Pay close attenion to how it seems immediately after the lochia bleeding stops. As long as the scant, stiff mucus stays exactly as it was at the early time (4-8 weeks after delivery) it can be considered infertile as if dry. Then you must watch carefully for any change at all toward the creamier, more abundant type of "early mucus" which will precede the wet fertile mucus. As soon as you notice an increase or change, you must consider it as "early mucus" and potentialy fertile. If you have mucus of any kind from then on, you must abstain for the duration of the mucus plus 3 dry days beyond. You are infertile on the 4th dry day.*

BE CAREFUL!
IF IN DOUBT,
DON'T DO IT.

1	2	3	4	5	6	⑦	8	9	10	11	12	13	14	⑮	16
dry	—	*creamy*	dry	dry	dry	—	*wet*	wet	wet	dry	dry	dry	dry		

*For the vast majority of women, any time during the 4th day is safe. But if you want the utmost in surety, you can add the extra 12 hours and wait until evening.

When your baby is about three or four months old, and sometimes earlier, you are likely to have "fertile mucus" every so often, which does not result in a period 5-12 days later. These were false alarem, and were not ovulation, or you would have gotten your period afterward. These false alarms are caused by your hormones trying to ovulate. Sometimes they came close, but didn't quite make it. The closer you get to that first ovulation, the more false alarms you are likely to have. Don't get frustrated and confused. One of these times it will be the real thing, and you will get a period 5-12 day later. Treat "false alarms" as if they are the real thing because one of them is, and at the time, you have no way of knowing which one it will be.

If you want infallible birth control in the post partum time, I suggest you abstain from making love until your periods return. There is a slight risk of pregnancy any time you make love before ovulation has passed (as demonstrated by a rise in temperature). If you are nursing often throughout the day and night, the risk is a lot less than if you introduce solid foods early and/or have the baby sleep through the night.

If you choose this conservative approach, you may be in for months of abstinence, But it's not really that long compared to the years ahead.

After childbirth, the first 2-3 cycles are often pretty irregular, with early or late ovulation, and consequently short or long cycles. So make love only during the first four days of your period, and after the temp rises later in the cycle.

Pay particularly close attention around the time of weaning, or any time—even temporary—when you cut back on nursing. If you or your baby are sick and you don't nurse as much, that could start your ovulation hormones working. You may ovulate at this time. A return to substantial nursing might stop the process; your mucus would dry up, and ovulation would not occur.

Special reminder: On days when you're supposed to abstain, don't make love using withdrawal, and don't get any seminal fluid anywhere near any mucus or near your vagina. One drop on the inside or outside can get you pregnant.

You may only have high temps for 5-10 days before the first period even though you usually have 10-16 days of high temps before most periods.

If you were already taking your temperature before the period began, and if this period was preceded by high temps, you can make love for the first 4 days and then wait for the T° to rise.

January

1	dry
②	dry
3	dry
④	dry
5	dry
⑥	dry
7	slightly wet
8	dry
9	dry
10	dry / pasty
⑪	dry
12	slightly wet
13	dry
14	dry
15	dry
⑯	dry
17	dry
18	dry
⑲	dry
20	dry
㉑	dry (tiny bit diff)
22	—
23	dry
24	slightly wet
25	dry
26	dry
27	dry
㉘	dry
29	dry
㉚	dry
31	dry

Here are some examples of Mucus Only Charts. You should make yourself nice charts like these and write it down every day. If you put value into your charts and keep them neat and highly detailed, they will serve you well. You may think you can keep it all in your head, but believe me, experience has shown that you will do much better if you take the time and energy to collect your data in an organized way.

This woman is in her third month after delivery. She is mostly dry with a little stiff, pasty mucus which has been the same since she quit bleeding. On days 7 and 12 and 24, she was slightly wet, probably due to making love the previous night. She abstained those nights and the three following nights just in case it was some mucus. Evidently it wasn't, because she was dry again right away.

80

May

Day	Observation
1	wet
2	wet
3	thin, white, milky
4	wet
5	spian
6	lots wet
7	wet
8	milky
9	lots milky
10	dry
11	scant tacky
12	wet
13	lots wet
14	less wet
15	dry
16	white milky
17	white milky
18	tacky
19	dry
20	scant wet
21	wet
22	white tacky
23	dry
24	sick wet
25	sick spian
26	lots wet
27	dry
28	wet
29	dry
30	tacky
31	wet

This couple wasn't able to make love all month long. She never had enough dry or infertile days in a row. This happens sometimes, especially when a woman is approaching her first ovulation and period. This is an opportunity to be creative with your loving, to be cooperative, and supportive of each other.

81

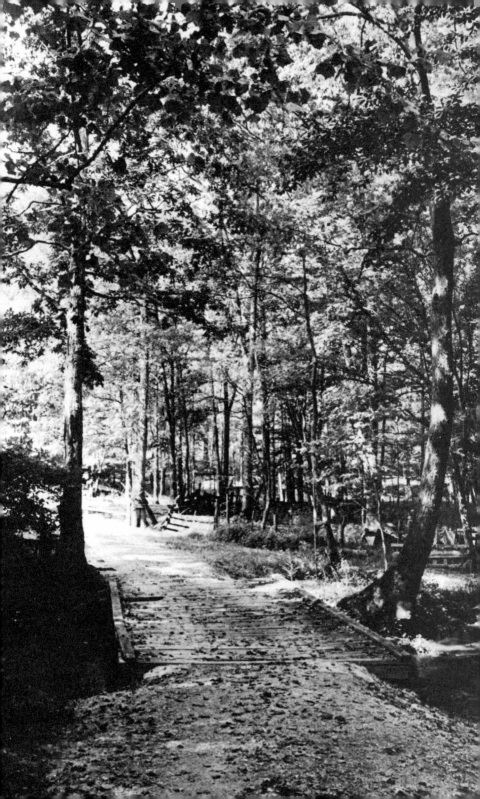

Menopause

Menopause is the tapering off of a woman's fertility. Ovulations, and therefore periods occur infrequently and farther apart until they stop altogether. It is very common to skip three or four ovulations and periods, and then ovulate and get a period two weeks later. You can think you are finished with periods and fertility for good, and then get yet one more. Or you may tend to spot (bleed a slight amount) often. Some spotting may be "breakthough bleeding" of ovulation, or it could be a scant period. If your temperature was high before the bleeding, it was a period. If it was low, it was not. Your cervical mucus will also still warn you of ovulation, no matter how infrequent, and you can check it with your temperature.

Even if you have periods irregularly, it's still a good idea to chart your BBT. For interpreting your mucus, follow the directions given for nursing mothers with no periods. You will probably not have the abundant mucus and "false alarms" that they have, so it should be easier for you.

> Do not make love until the fourth day past any spotting because it could be ovulation rather than a period.

You will probably be "dry" most of the time, except when ovulation is approaching, and if you chart your temperature and mucus every day faithfully, you will certainly notice a build-up of mucus that forewarns ovulation, and a temperature rise that confirms it.

After "The Pill"

If you are just coming off the pill, you should be very cautious for the first few months. You may find yourself skipping periods, or extra fertile. When you take birth control pills, you don't have true periods. You have what's called "withdrawal bleeding" caused by stopping the pill each month for a few days. So, when you quit taking pills, your whole system has to readjust to a natural cycle. Your mucus may not be accurate for a few months as the hormones readjust. So, rely on your BBT chart and make love only after the rise in temperature for a few months. Observe and chart everything, but act only on the results of your temperature chart. You will have to start fresh in gathering cycle length data for your calendar rhythm calculations, since the cycle-length on pills is not your real cycle length. Read the section on "Basal Body Temperature" very carefully and don't rely on calendar rhythm or mucus observations for any early safe time for a few months.

If You Wish To Conceive

If you are trying to have a baby, and perhaps it has been difficult in the past, the principles in this book might help you conceive. I certainly hope so. Basically, you will need to follow the rules herein backwards. Read this whole book carefully so you understand the principles of fertility. Chart your temperature and your mucus in order to find out if and when you ovulate. If you have a temperature chart that goes from low readings to high readings, you are ovulating. Watch your mucus for Spinn., as it will indicate your maximum day of fertility. It would be a good idea for you and your husband to avoid making love for about five days before you expect to ovulate in order for him to have a high sperm count. This will be during the time your mucus is building up in quantity and becoming clearer. When you observe Spinn., make love once. Then skip a day and make love again as your temperature begins to ascend. The day of Spinn. is usually the day before ovulation, and is the most fertile day of your cycle. If you make love then, you will have fresh young sperm waiting for the egg to emerge. You then skip a day to allow your husband to build up some more sperm, and try again one more time before the egg passes on. After that you can make love freely until about five days before you next expect to ovulate. These five days will usually correspond to the days of increasing fertile mucus. If you do not get any Spinn. (some women don't), then use the day of maximum clear mucus. Incidentally, your husband should avoid hot baths as this can lower his sperm count. Sperm don't do well when the surrounding temperature is quite hot. A hot shower if fine, but have him avoid hot baths while you are trying to conceive. Best of luck to you.

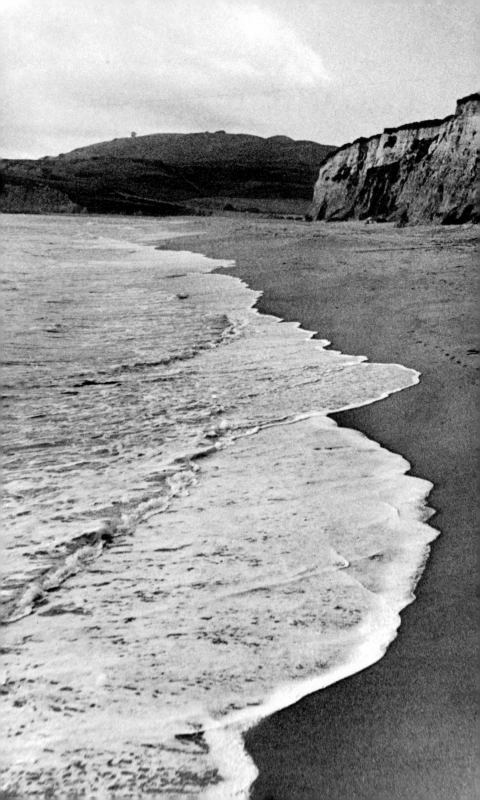

CHANGES OF THE CERVIX

There is one more sign of fertility that you might want to check along with the others. This is the cervix exam. It is completely optional, and you can practice natural family planning quite well without it, if it does not appeal to you. The cervix exam can be especially helpful during nursing or pre-menopause, and for women with long cycles.

If you remember, the cervix of the uterus is the narrow, lower part of the uterus that fits into the top of the vaginal canal and produces fertile mucus when the hormone estrogen is high. In addition to producing cervical mucus, the cervix itself goes through changes each month as estrogen rises and falls:

1.) It changes elevation (along with entire uterus) in the abdomen. It actually goes up and down as the uterine ligaments get tighter and looser on a hormonal schedule.

2.) It becomes softer or harder to the touch, and

3.) the size of the tiny opening changes

The cervix is low in the vaginal canal (easy to reach), with a tilt toward the back wall of the vagina, during the infertile part of the cycle. It moves higher (harder to reach), and lies straighter in the canal, during the fertile days surrounding ovulation.

As ovulation approaches, the cervix begins to soften, like the texture of your lips. The os gradually opens over the course of about five days. The cervix rises up in the body and becomes harder to reach. This happens at the same time as the beginning of the mucus discharge. Just before ovulation the tiny opening will be large enough that your finger tip can slide into it about 1/4 to 1/2 inch. The cervix will feel soft and wet with fertile mucus.

After ovulation has come and gone, the os closes and the cervix feels firm and rather dry, like the tip of your nose. At this infertile time the os will contain a plug of thick mucus which protects the uterus from the outside world during most of the cycle. The closed os feels like a dimple and your finger will not be able to enter.

A good time to perform the exam is in the morning, perhaps at your first visit to the bathroom. Be sure your fingernails and hands are washed. Stand with your back curled forward and one foot on a stool or chair. Reach one or two fingers toward your backbone to find it. If you cannot reach it, try pressing your abdomen down from above with the other hand.

When you find the cervix, feel for firmness or softness, the size of the opening, and highness or lowness in the abdomen. Before withdrawing your fingers, if you wish, you can collect some mucus at the source.

The cervix sign is not to be used alone. It should be used to confirm the other major signs. And if your cervix suggests you might be fertile when other signs are borderline, heed the warning. Mark different sized little circles and a few descriptive words in the space for "other comments" on your chart.

Again, this special sign is not necessary to the practice of natural birth control, but it can be very helpful if you are inclined to use it.

The changes of the cervix were originally documented by Dr. Edward F. Keefe (Keefe EF. Physicians help make rhythm work. NY State J Med 1976;76:205-208).

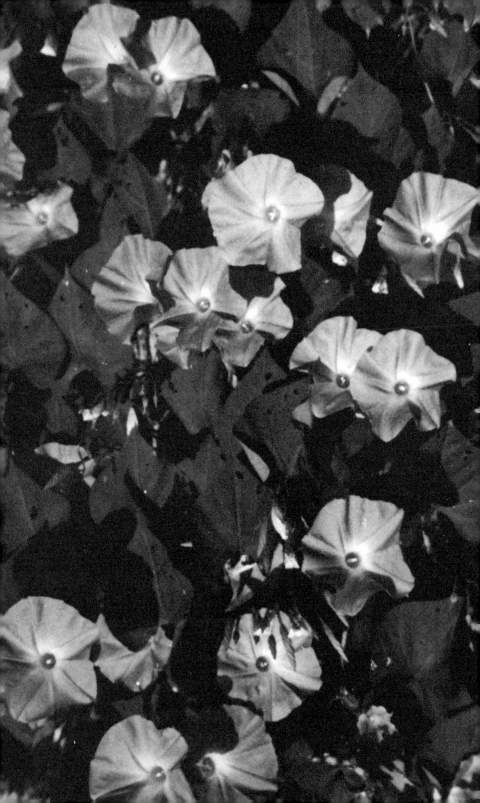

QUESTIONS
&
ANSWERS

Q. I have lots of fertile looking mucus late in my cycle, after ovulation seems to be over. It starts about a week or 10 days past my ovulation mucus. Am I possibly ovulating twice?

A. No, you are not ovulating twice in one cycle, unless it is within a few hours with fraternal twins. That fertile looking mucus late in your cycle is a result of hormone changes leading to your period. Your BBT also falls a few days before your period. The hormone that keeps your BBT high and your mucus scant starts to fade a few days before your period.

Q. My temperature jumps around quite a bit in the first half of my cycle, before ovulation. Once I ovulate, it gets high and stays there, but I wondered about that first part.

A. It's quite all right for your temperature to be a little wild in the early segment of your cycle. Some women's temperatures stay low at this time and some go up and down. But you will find that in general, the temperatures before ovulation are lower than those after ovulation.

Q. I get a lot of mucus before I make love when I've been dry all day. Is this fertile mucus?

A. It may be fertile mucus from your cervix or it may be from the lubricating glands right inside your vagina. If you check your mucus when you are ready to make love, it may be the lubricating mucus. But if you check in the evening before you are even thinking about making love, and it is wet and slippery, it is probably fertile mucus from your cervix. If there is any doubt at all, don't do it.

Q. I would like to take my temperature at the same time each morning, but I have to get up with my nursing baby at night and in the early morning hours. What should I do?

A. Pick the time when you get the longest period of sleep. Then take your temperature at that time every morning. If your baby wakes up at 4:00 or 5:00 each morning, use him for your alarm clock. Ask your husband to bring him to you while you take your temperature. Try to get at least three hours of sleep before taking your temperature, and try to take it around the same time each morning. But if you only got one hour of sleep one night, or if you are taking it at a vastly different time than usual, take it anyway and note an explanation on your chart. Don't ever skip a day of taking your temperature because of odd circumstances. It's better to have a reading with an explanation than nothing at all.

Q. I am nursing and have no periods yet, so I am relying on my mucus changes to warn me of my first ovulation. But sometimes I am so wet so much of the time that my husband and I can't make love for weeks at a time. What should I do?

A. Your hormones are so active at this time that they keep giving you "false alarms" of ovulation. This usually happens for a month or two before your first ovulation and period. For a few women, it can go on for several months. You and your husband need to be patient and extra good to each other. It may seem like a long time but it is really very short compared to the years ahead of you once you re-establish your cycles.

Q. Is there any reason why my husband and I shouldn't use "withdrawal" during my fertile times?

A. (Withdrawal is when a couple makes love until right before his orgasm, at which time he withdraws.) Withdrawal is not a good idea for two reasons. First of all, your husband can lose a drop of semen before orgasm and the first few drops have the most sperm in them. Second (but of equal importance), it will probably drive your husband crazy after a while. The stakes are too high and he won't be able to relax.

Q. I had two children right in a row and never had a period in between. How was that possible?

A. You got pregnant the first time you ovulated after your first child. You would have gotten your period two weeks later if you had not gotten pregnant.

Q. I am in menopause and sometimes don't have a period for several months. What should I do?

A. If you don't have a period very often, then you are not ovulating very often, either. You can depend on your cervical mucus to warn you of ovulation when it does come. Read all the sections in this book that pertain to mucus and chart your mucus changes faithfully. Then you will know when ovulation approaches and you are fertile. Birth control need not be a problem during menopause.

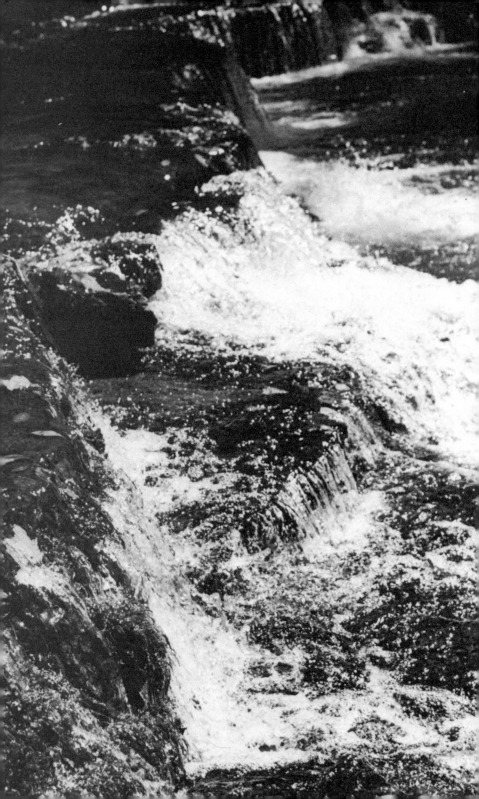

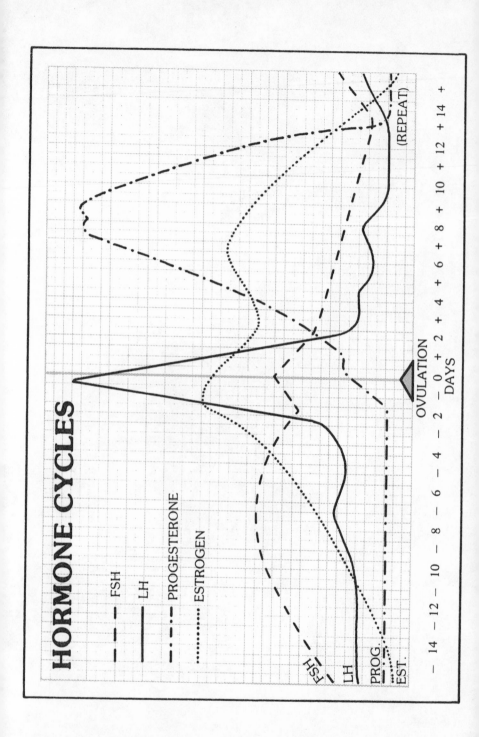

HORMONE CYCLES

FSH
LH
PROGESTERONE
ESTROGEN

OVULATION

DAYS

− 14 − 12 − 10 − 8 − 6 − 4 − 2 − 0 + 2 + 4 + 6 + 8 + 10 + 12 + 14 +

(REPEAT)

FSH
LH
PROG.
EST.

96

Female Endocrinology

To accomplish this natural method of birth control, it helps quite a lot to understand the *natural mechanisms of your fertility cycle*. These natural methods proceed out of scientific principles of female physiology and endocrinology. *You don't need to memorize all of this to practice natural birth control, but you really should have some idea of what's happening.*

The hormones involved in the female reproductive cycle are all interdependent and operate through feedback mechanisms among each other. Science isn't yet sure of the exact order of the feedback mechanisms. (Which came first, the chicken or the egg?) But this is more or less what the picture looks like:

The endocrine hormones that determine your cycle come from the anterior (front) portion of the pituitary gland (which is in the center of your head) and from the ovaries themselves.

Pituitary Hormones

FSH - Follicle Stimulating Hormone—causes the egg to ripen and mature.

LH - Luteinizing Hormone—causes further ripening of the egg, ovulation, and the formation of the corpus luteum (the endocrine gland created from the burst follicle.)

Ovarian Hormones

Estrogen - Basic female hormone whch maintains female characteristics and helps regulate the release of FSH and LH.

Progesterone - The hyperthermic (heat producing hormone) secreted from the corpus luteum. Along with estrogen, it prepares the uterine lining to receive a fertilized egg, and prevents the loss of this lining if a fertilized egg implants in it.

The anterior pituitary starts the process by secreting the

Follicle Stimulating Hormone

— FSH —

It is influenced to do this by Gonadotropin Releasing Hormone (GnRH) from a portion of the brain called the *hypothalamus*. The hypothalamus signals the pituitary to secrete FSH (and a little LH) which starts a cluster of follicles in the ovary maturing.

When FSH travels through the bloodstream and hits the ovary, it causes the follicles that are beginning to ripen to secrete *another* hormone -

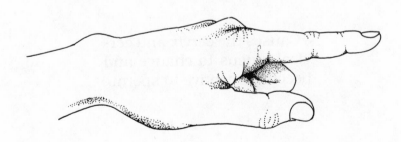

-- Estrogen --

As the follicles ripen over a period of about seven days, they secrete more and more estrogen into the bloodstream. Estrogen causes many things to happen.

It:

- Causes the womb to begin preparing its lining to possibly receive and nourish a baby.

- Causes the cervix and cervical mucus to change and become receptive to sperm.

The sharp midcycle rise in estrogen causes a surge in -

-- LH --

This sharp rise in LH causes ovulation of the ripest egg from the group of eggs that have matured under the influence of FSH.

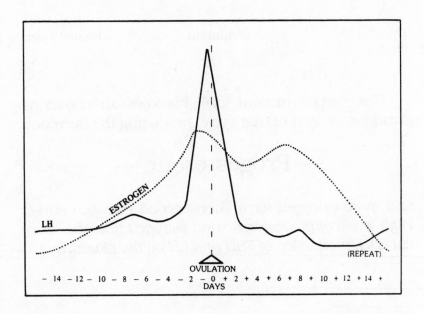

Then LH causes the empty follicle, the crater where the egg was, to be transformed into the

— Corpus Luteum —

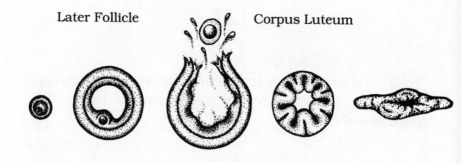

Later Follicle   Corpus Luteum

Early   Ovulation   Healed Over
Follicle

The corpus luteum itself becomes an endocrine gland for the rest of that cycle, producing the hormone

— Progesterone —

and more estrogen for a short second estrogen surge. *High levels of progesterone and estrogen from the ovary cut back production of FSH and LH by the pituitary.*

After ovulation, the *follicular phase* of the cycle, designated by *high estrogen* levels, ends. The *luteal phase*, with *high progesterone* levels, begins.

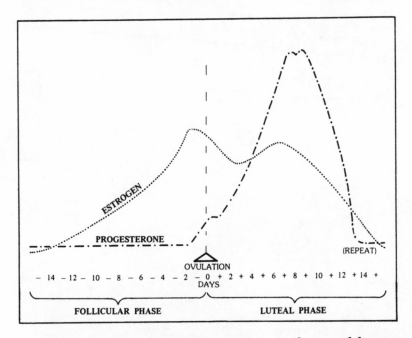

The main job of progesterone is to thoroughly prepare the lining of the womb, finishing the job started by estrogen.

The lining of the womb builds up rapidly. The luteal phase lasts about two weeks (12-16 days). Then the corpus luteum stops producing progesterone and scars over. When the progesterone level in the blood falls, the womb sheds its lining. At this point, pituitary FSH comes back into prominence and the cycle starts over again.

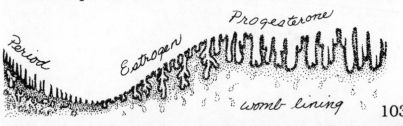

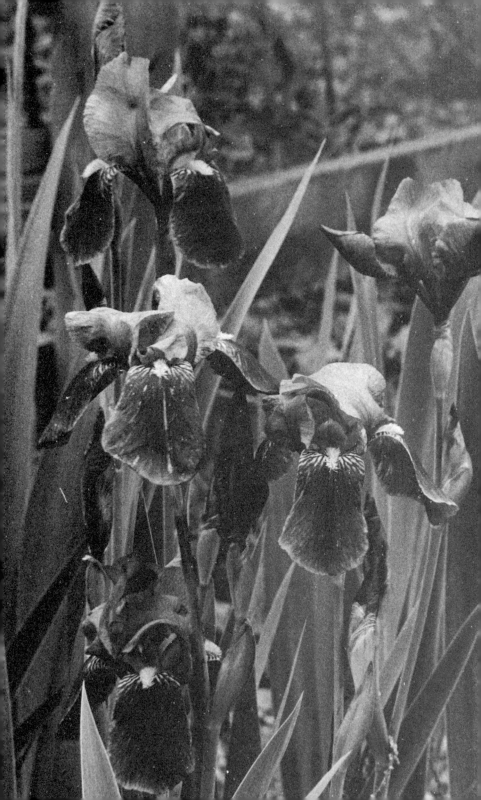

Yeast
and
Other Vaginal Infections

There are three common female infections that can interfere with the interpretation of cervical mucus. These are *Candida albicans* (monilia), commonly known as "yeast"; bacterial overgrowth or infection; and a protozoa called *Trichomonas*.

Yeast is the most common and least serious. Yeast is a fungus that causes itching and burning, and produces a curdy, white discharge which does not have a bad odor. Having monilla is like having tiny mushroom colonies in your vaginal canal. Don't make love while you have a yeast infection because it makes it worse by breaking it up and spreading the yeast colonies. The effective medications have changed from prescription to over-the-counter status, and you can now treat yourself without a doctor visit. Sometimes a very mild yeast problem can be treated with a douche of 2 TBSP vinegar to a quart of warm water.

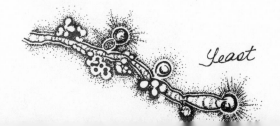

Yeast

If you have vaginal itching with no burning, and your discharge is profuse and slightly foamy with a bad odor, you probably have Trichomonas. This is a protozoan infection which is carried by men and women, but usually only symptomatic in women. You must see your doctor for Trichomonas because he or she will treat you and your mate with metronidazole tablets, which are only sold by prescription.

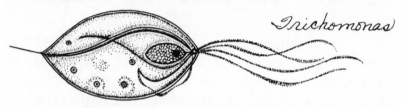

Trichomonas

If you have a vaginal discharge that does not itch, but may be irritating, and has an unpleasant odor, you probably have a bacterial infection. Again, you will need to see your doctor, as he or she will treat you with prescription drugs and/or creams or suppositories.

In general, it is not a good idea to douche unless you are treating a yeast infection. Your vaginal canal is self-cleaning. If you douche often, you can upset the delicate balance of microorganisms that naturally reside in the vagina.

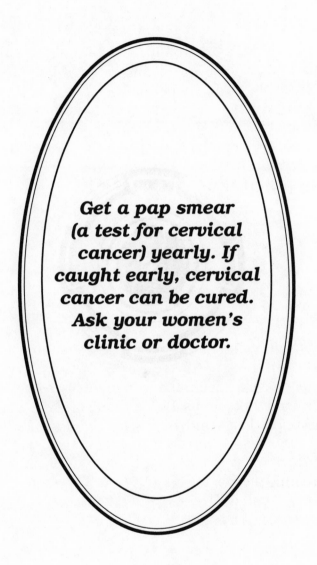

*Get a pap smear
(a test for cervical
cancer) yearly. If
caught early, cervical
cancer can be cured.
Ask your women's
clinic or doctor.*

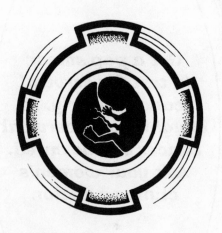

INDEX

BASAL TEMPERATURE AND MUCUS CHART

MONTH _____ thru _____

Date																																								
Day of week M.T.W.Th.etc.																																								
Day of cycle	1	2	3	4	5	6	7	8	9	10	11	12	13	14	15	16	17	18	19	20	21	22	23	24	25	26	27	28	29	30	31	32	33	34	35	36	37	38	39	40

Temp.

.5
.4
.3
.2
.1
99.0
.9
.8
.7
.6
.5
.4
.3
.2
.1
98.0
.9
.8
.7
.6
.5
.4
.3
.2
.1
97.0

Place a dot in the center of the square under the day and across from the temperature. Connect the dots with straight lines.

mucus

Use several descriptive words such as: creamy, wet, white, clear, sticky, slippery, spinn, milky, scant, cloudy, lots, pink, stiff, translucent

Ovulation Pain-Pressure

comment

Any notable circumstances fever, illness, travel, stress, lack of sleep, emotional, etc

Number of days in this cycle: _____

Shortest previous cycle: _____

111

You can order the following books directly from:

THE BOOK PUBLISHING COMPANY
PO Box 99
Summertown, TN 38483

A Cooperative Method of Natural Birth Control	$6.95
In the Newborn Year:	
Our Changing Awareness After Childbirth	$9.95
Physician's Slimming Guide	$5.95
The Power of Your Plate	$10.95
Spiritual Midwifery (Third Edition)	$16.95
Why Not Me? The Story of Gladys Milton, Midwife	$9.95

Please inlude $2. per book additional for shipping.

If you are interested in other fine books on alternative health, ecology, vegetarian cooking, gardening, Native Americans and children's books, **CALL FOR A CATALOG 800-695-2241**